S0-ESC-720

FAQ

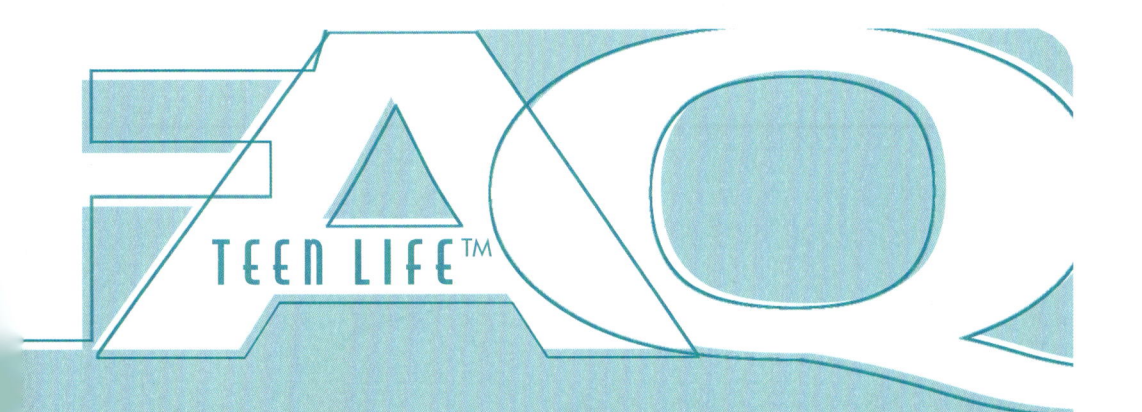

TEEN LIFE™

FREQUENTLY ASKED QUESTIONS ABOUT

Human Papillomavirus

Lissette Gonzalez

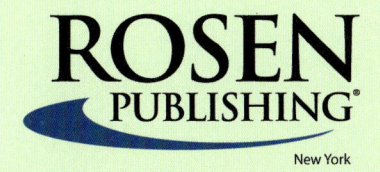

RosenPublishing®
New York

Published in 2009 by The Rosen Publishing Group, Inc.
29 East 21st Street, New York, NY 10010

Copyright © 2009 by The Rosen Publishing Group, Inc.

First Edition

All rights reserved. No part of this book may be reproduced in any form without permission in writing from the publisher, except by a reviewer.

Library of Congress Cataloging-in-Publication Data

Gonzalez, Lissette, 1968–
Frequently asked questions about human papillomavirus / Lissette Gonzalez.
   p. cm.—(FAQ: teen life)
ISBN-13: 978-1-4042-1813-0 (library binding)
1. Papillomavirus diseases. I. Title.
RC168.P15G66 2007
616.9'11—dc22

2008010302

Manufactured in the United States of America

Contents

1 What Is Human Papillomavirus? 4

2 What Are the Symptoms of Human Papillomavirus and How Is It Diagnosed? 9

3 How Can Human Papillomavirus Be Prevented? 16

4 What Are the Treatment Options for Human Papillomavirus? 28

5 What Is the Connection Between Human Papillomavirus and Cervical Cancer? 34

6 What Is the Connection Between Human Papillomavirus and Penile and Anal Cancers? 45

Glossary 55
For More Information 58
For Further Reading 61
Index 62

Chapter one

WHAT IS HUMAN PAPILLOMAVIRUS?

Every year in the United States, three million teenagers contract some type of sexually transmitted disease, or STD. While most think it will never happen to them, studies from the Alan Guttmacher Institute and the Kaiser Family Foundation reveal that about one in four American teens becomes infected.

According to the American Social Health Association (ASHA), the most common STD in the United States today is a group of viruses known as human papillomavirus, or HPV. The number of new HPV infections in the United States is an estimated five and a half million every year. HPV has become so widespread that as many as twenty million people are believed to have an active genital HPV infection at any point in time.

If you've never heard of HPV before, you're not alone. ASHA's background report on HPV points out that in one

WHAT IS HUMAN PAPILLOMAVIRUS?

Below is a papillomavirus as seen through an electron microscope.

national survey, 76 percent of female respondents were completely unaware of HPV.

If you are a teenager and are reading about HPV for the first time, you may rightly wonder what this means to you, where you can go for more information, and what steps you can take to protect your health. STDs such as HPV are sometimes difficult to talk about. Teens are often embarrassed because of the stigma associated with STDs. It is very important to address this subject, however, since many STDs, including HPV, may have no obvious symptoms. If you are not aware of the facts, it is often difficult to tell if you're in need of treatment or if you have been infected. In fact, one reason HPV and other STDs are so easily spread is that a lot of people don't even know that they are infected, and they infect others without realizing it.

Learning about HPV is a valuable first step toward overcoming any awkwardness you may feel about STDs. It will also help you make responsible decisions about your health and sexual behavior.

HPV Defined

Human papillomavirus, or HPV, is a group of viruses that cause an infection that affects the skin and mucous membranes of the body. A virus is a microscopic organism made up of protein and genetic material (DNA). Viruses are so small that they can only be seen with very powerful tools called electron microscopes. Viruses can get into the body when it comes into contact with the body of an infected person. In the case of HPV, one person can give the virus to another during sex or other types of activities. Once inside the body, viruses multiply by making copies of themselves.

HPV actually refers to a group of about one hundred different viruses. About one-third of the known HPV viruses are sexually transmitted. HPV is sometimes called the wart virus because it is most often associated with the warts that some strains can cause on the genitals or on other parts of the body.

It is more common for people to develop HPV without symptoms than it is for them to exhibit signs of genital warts. HPV infections that can cause warts—whether hidden or obvious—are classified as low-risk infections because they usually do not lead to cancer. Other higher-risk strains of HPV (strains 16, 18, 31, 33, and 45 of the virus), while not likely ever to cause genital warts, are linked to certain cancers in females and other cancers in males. For example, certain strains of HPV are now known to be the leading cause of cancer of the cervix (the portion of the uterus that opens into the vagina) in females. HPV is also linked to cancer of the penis in males and to cancer of the anus in both males and females.

> Also known as wart virus, human papillomavirus can result in warts such as the one pictured here.

When HPV develops into genital warts (also known as venereal warts), the growths can grow on, in, or around the anus, inside the vagina, or on the penis. Genital warts may also appear on the outer pubic skin, the groin area, and the areas near the inner thigh. In some cases, genital warts can become quite large and grow to resemble cauliflower. However, this is not always the case, and warts may be overlooked if they are very small, flat, flesh-colored, or painless. Symptoms such as itching, bleeding, or pain are not common but can occur.

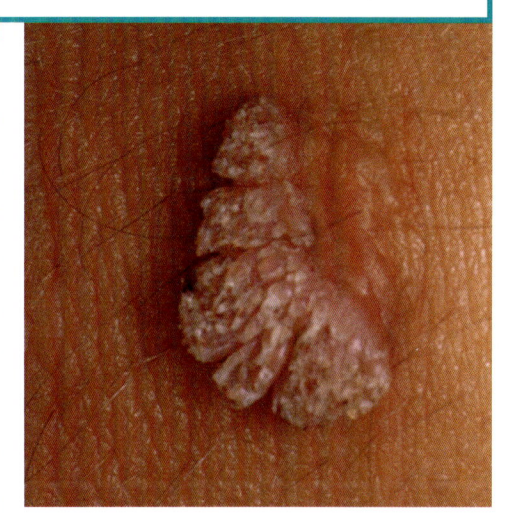

Although genital warts are an obvious sign of HPV infection, many who contract HPV never develop genital warts. In fact, most people who become infected with HPV don't even know they have it. This is because the body's immune system holds HPV at bay, leaving no visible symptoms, even though the infection is still present within the body. This means that although you have no symptoms or wart growths, you could still infect others with HPV. This also means that you can be infected by your partner even if he or she shows no visible signs of HPV infection.

The strains of HPV that lead to genital warts are different from those that produce warts on the hands and feet.

What Exactly Are Warts?

A wart is a rough round or oval raised overgrowth of skin caused by HPV, an infection in the top layer of the skin. There are several types of warts. Each has a different appearance, depending on where it grows.

Warts have an interesting history and have been written about for centuries. Known to the Romans as *verrucas*, genital warts were suspected to be sexually transmitted as far back as 25 CE. The suggestion that warts were caused by a virus came much later, in nineteenth-century England. It was only after 1950, however, when papillomavirus particles were finally analyzed under a microscope, that scientists accepted the virus connection.

Many people still remain confused about HPV and warts, how the virus is contracted, how it is spread, and how it develops in the body. In an effort to share accurate information with the public, health-care providers, and others, ASHA has recently set up the National HPV and Cervical Cancer Prevention Resource Center, which has a toll-free HPV hotline: (800) 227-8922. In addition to the most up-to-date information on HPV and cancer prevention, the center also provides lists of community resources and support groups for those dealing with the emotional issues that follow the discovery of genital HPV or cancer.

chapter two

WHAT ARE THE SYMPTOMS OF HUMAN PAPILLOMAVIRUS AND HOW IS IT DIAGNOSED?

Genital warts and other strains of human papillomavirus (HPV) are spread through skin-to-skin contact during anal, oral, or vaginal sex with an infected person. HPV and genital warts can infect any sexually active teenager or adult. You can have sex with someone and not know that you've become infected with HPV or genital warts. This is because genital warts don't always appear quickly; in some instances, people infected with HPV don't develop any symptoms at all. HPV can live in the skin and body without any warts or changes occurring. This is called latent (hidden) HPV. You can still infect others with HPV and genital warts when you have no symptoms.

In other cases, symptoms may occur weeks, months, or years after becoming infected. Usually, however, genital warts develop between three and eight months after exposure.

Once a person is infected, HPV could lead to the following results:

- **Latent or inactive infection:** Infected areas appear to be normal because the body's immune system is controlling the virus. Even though you can't see any changes, you may still infect others during vaginal, oral, or anal sex.
- **Subclinical or active infection I:** HPV begins to cause cellular changes inside the body, which in females are sometimes seen as "abnormal" results on a Pap smear. (A Pap smear is a quick, painless test that allows doctors to collect a very small tissue sample from a female's cervix.) These abnormal cellular changes sometimes lead to the development of cancer in both males and females.
- **Clinical or active infection II:** HPV begins to cause visible changes on the outside of the body in the form of genital warts. Genital warts do not lead to cancer, but their presence should alert both you and your doctor to do further testing to determine if cancer is present in the body.

Symptoms of Genital Warts

Genital (venereal) warts can appear on the penis, the vulva, or the opening of the anus. They may also develop inside the vagina, throat, or anus. They may be small or large, flat or

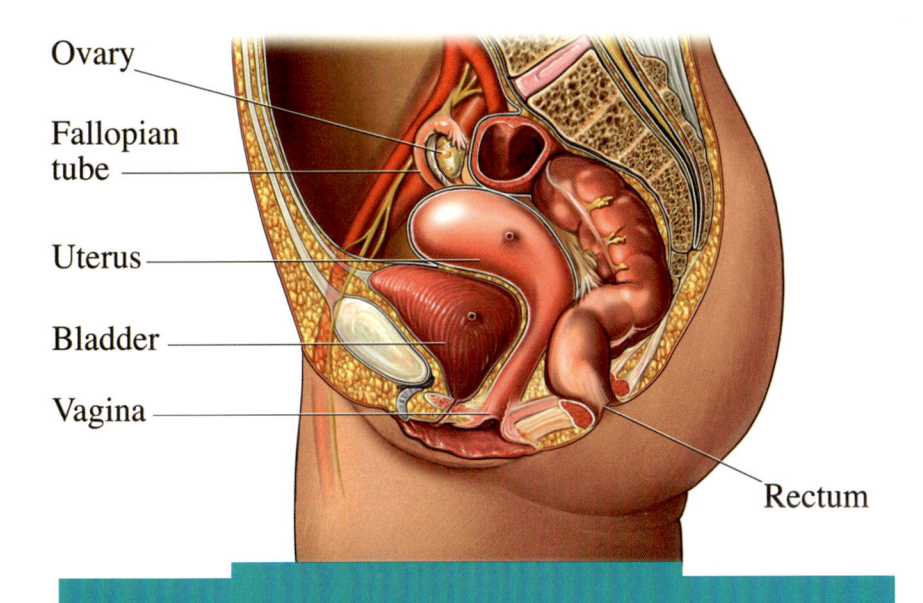

WHAT ARE THE SYMPTOMS OF HUMAN PAPILLOMAVIRUS AND HOW IS IT DIAGNOSED?

Above is a diagram of the female reproductive system.

raised, single or in clusters resembling cauliflower. They may also be in more than one area of the body and often develop on pubic skin, an area that condoms don't cover. This is why it is important to look at your own body, as well as your partner's, before becoming intimate. For both teens and adults, speaking frankly, openly, and honestly about STDs and their prevention is a prerequisite to any responsible sexual activity. Young women should make their first visit to a gynecologist after they begin to menstruate and before they become sexually active. A gynecologist is a doctor who specializes in diseases of and the care of the female reproductive organs.

Any unusual growths or changes on your skin or the skin of anyone you've had sex with should be examined by a doctor, especially if you suspect you've been infected with genital warts or any other STD.

While genital warts are not life threatening, their discovery can be very frightening. It is common to feel angry with the person who you believe infected you. You may feel alone or ashamed. Remember, genital warts can be successfully treated.

Diagnosing Genital Warts

If you are female, your doctor or nurse may use a special magnifying lens called a colposcope to clearly see warts in the cervix or other places inside the body. This test is called a colposcopy. Another method of detection for both males and females involves placing a vinegar preparation on the genitals and other affected areas. This turns any warts that are present white, making them easier to see and therefore treat.

For many young women, a Pap smear will show the first presence of a potential HPV infection. A Pap smear is the microscopic examination of cells carefully swabbed from the inside of a female's vagina or cervix.

When the results of a regular Pap smear screening are "positive" or abnormal, the doctor will examine the cervix further to determine if the HPV infection is present. An abnormal Pap smear result could also indicate other conditions besides HPV infection.

Any abnormal results of a Pap smear screening could result in the doctor wanting to perform another smear for comparison

WHAT ARE THE SYMPTOMS OF HUMAN PAPILLOMAVIRUS AND HOW IS IT DIAGNOSED?

A cytobrush is one tool often used to take sample cells from a woman's cervix for a Pap smear.

or a test called a biopsy. A biopsy is the removal of a very small piece of tissue from inside the body. After the tissue is removed, it is tested for any other abnormalities, such as specific strains of the HPV infection. Some of these strains, especially those that show no visible genital warts, such as strains 16, 18, 31, 33, and 45, are now known to frequently cause cancer.

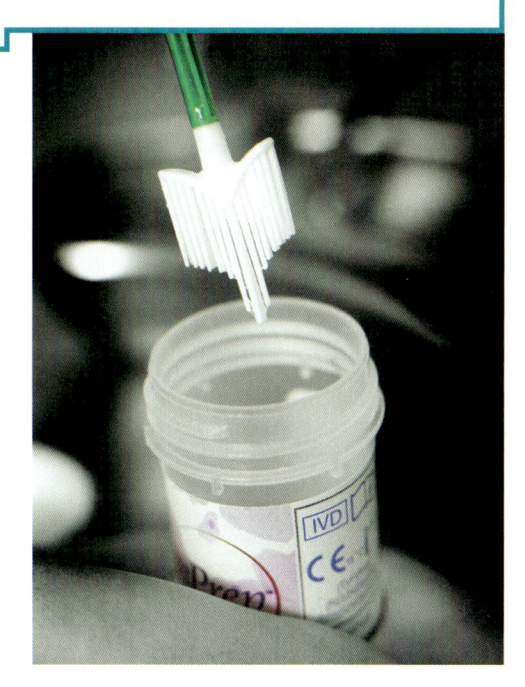

If genital warts are diagnosed, the doctor will discuss treatment options. The treatment he or she recommends will depend on several factors, including the size, sites, and number of warts to be treated.

What If You Are Pregnant?

Tell the doctor or nurse if you are pregnant and seeking treatment for genital warts. He or she can help you select a treatment that won't hurt you or your baby.

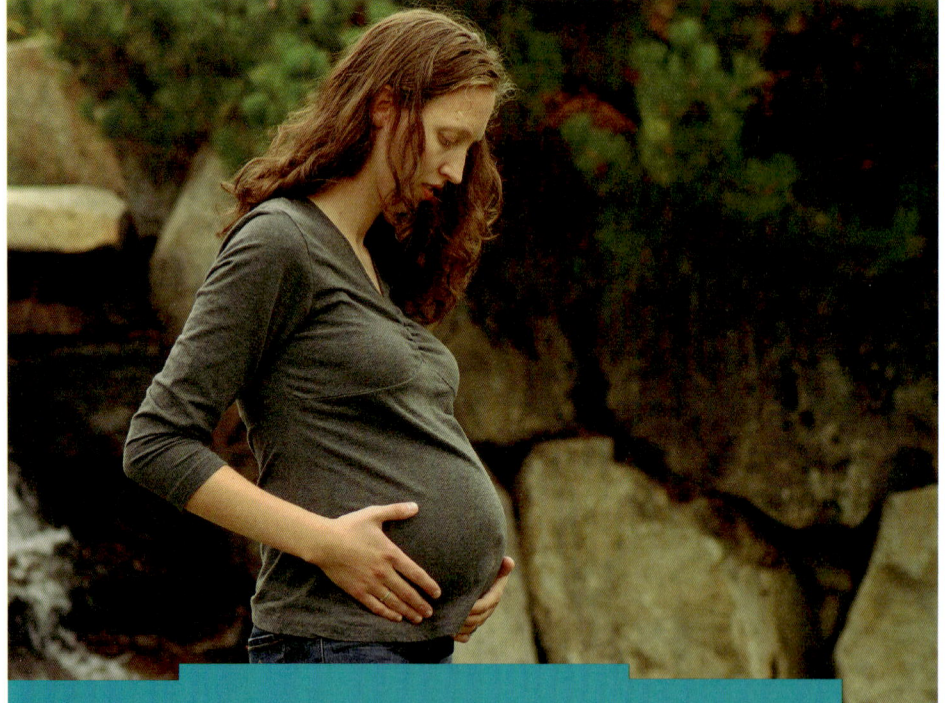

Being pregnant can aggravate any genital warts that are already present, causing them to grow larger. But genital warts are unlikely to cause any abnormalities in a pregnancy or birth.

According to the American Social Health Association, females with genital warts generally have normal pregnancies and births. While genital warts can be transmitted from mother to baby during the birthing process, this doesn't happen often and can be managed and treated if it occurs.

When you are pregnant, your body and hormones (the chemicals that regulate many of the body's functions) go through many changes. If you have genital warts, they may grow larger as a result of this increase in hormonal activity. You

WHAT ARE THE SYMPTOMS OF HUMAN PAPILLOMAVIRUS AND HOW IS IT DIAGNOSED?

may develop more of them than you would if you were not pregnant. If you have had genital warts in the past, and have been treated prior to becoming pregnant, it is unusual for them to return during your pregnancy.

Chapter three

HOW CAN HUMAN PAPILLOMAVIRUS BE PREVENTED?

HPV is quickly and easily passed from partner to partner through sexual contact. The sex organs are likely to be the first areas in which any symptoms appear; others are the mouth, throat, and anus.

HPV and Other STDs

It is important to know that if you have been infected with any other STD, such as chlamydia, hepatitis B or C, genital herpes, HIV/AIDS, gonorrhea, and/or syphilis, it is easier for strains of HPV to invade your body. The reason for this is that the body's immune system may not be able to combat more than one infection.

Once HPV has infected the body, it will remain in the cells for an indefinite time, most often in an invisible or latent stage. Still, latent HPV is able to produce symptoms whenever the body's immune system is slowed or compromised. Many situations could cause a recurrence of latent HPV, such as:

- Use of certain medications
- HIV infection
- Temporary trauma
- Serious illnesses
- Surgery
- Excessive stress

Hope to Prevent HPV

In June 2006, there was an exciting breakthrough in the medical community. A vaccine was approved by the Food and Drug Administration (FDA) that protects against four types of HPV. There is now a safe, effective new tool that girls and women can use to help protect themselves from HPV-related conditions. The vaccine is still relatively new, so more time and testing will be required to fully understand its potential, but the findings so far are incredibly promising. Here's what you need to know about the vaccine, what it does, and what it doesn't do, so you can talk with your parents and doctor to find out more about the vaccine.

Gardasil

The FDA approved Gardasil on June 8, 2006. The vaccine protects against HPV types 6, 11, 16, and 18. These are the types of HPV that cause 70 percent of cervical cancers and 90 percent of genital warts. Studies in young women have shown that there are no

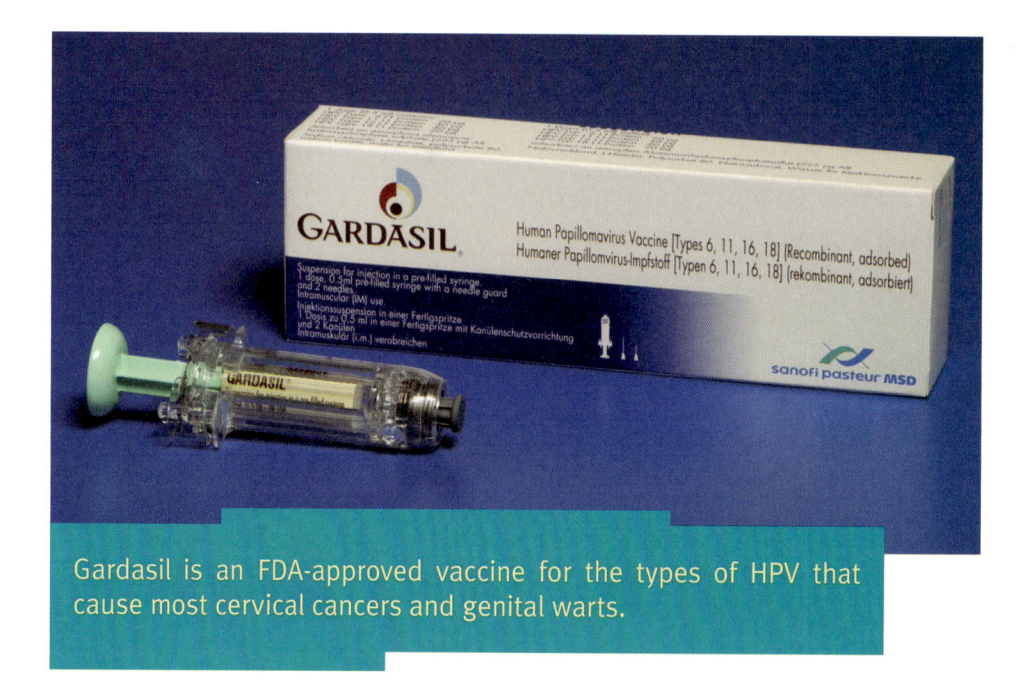

Gardasil is an FDA-approved vaccine for the types of HPV that cause most cervical cancers and genital warts.

serious side effects to the vaccine. The most common complaint was minor pain at the site of the injection. (The vaccine is injected into the muscle.)

Who Should Get the Vaccine?

The medical community is currently recommending that girls and women ages eleven to twenty-six get the vaccine. Some health professionals think it makes sense for girls as young as age nine to be vaccinated.

When Should You Get the Vaccine?

The best time to get the vaccine is before you have been sexually active because the vaccine works best if you have not acquired the HPV types the vaccine protects against. But even if you are, or have been, sexually active, the vaccine can still protect you from HPV types you have not acquired. Because there is no test to determine which HPV types a woman may or may not have in her body, it is probably a good idea to get the vaccine to be on the safe side.

What Does the Vaccine Do?

Studies have proven that the vaccine is 100 percent effective in preventing cervical precancers caused by HPV types 6, 11, 16, and 18. Precancers are abnormal cells that can, over time, turn into cancer. The vaccine has also been shown to be almost 100 percent effective in preventing genital warts and precancers of the vagina and vulva (the area outside the vagina).

What Doesn't the Vaccine Do?

The vaccine does not prevent a disease that could develop from a type of HPV a female already has. And the vaccine does not treat HPV-related diseases that a female already has. The vaccine does not prevent other sexually transmitted infections (STIs).

What Is Important to Remember?

The HPV vaccine is a breakthrough in preventing some HPV-related diseases, but it is not a replacement for cervical cancer screenings, or Pap smears, which help identify precancerous cells or other abnormalities in the cervix. The vaccine also cannot and should not replace safe, responsible sexual behavior, if you are, or are thinking about becoming, sexually active. It is

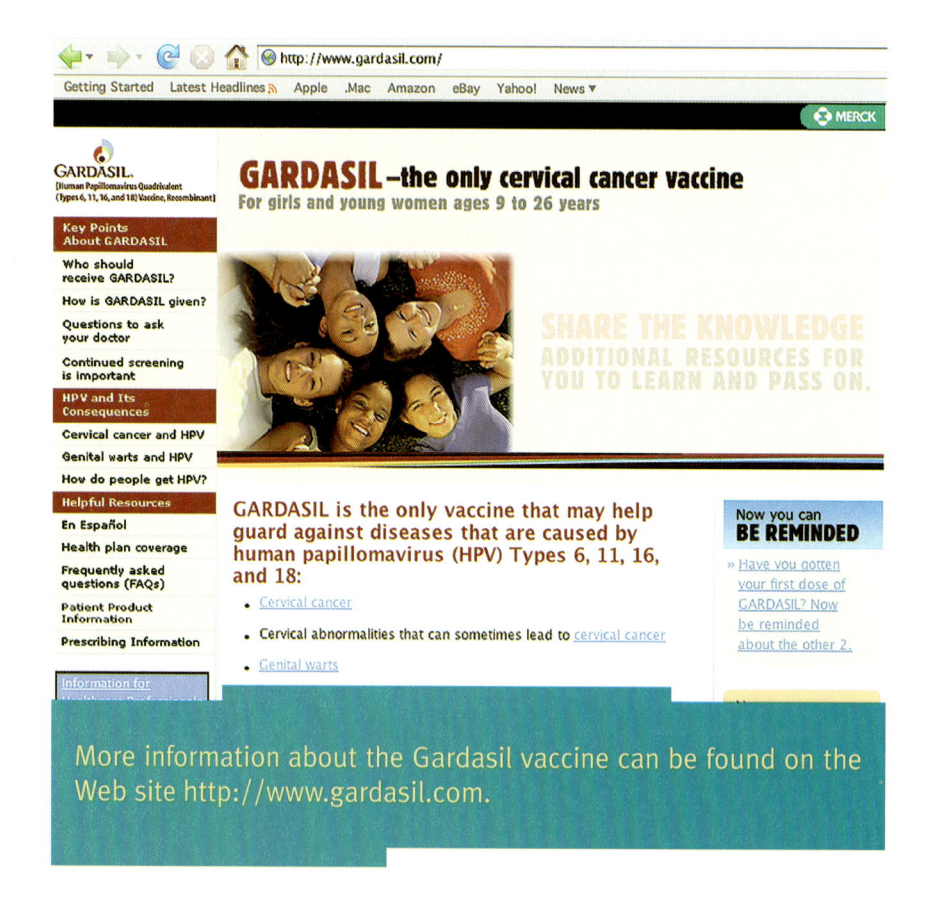

FREQUENTLY ASKED QUESTIONS ABOUT HUMAN PAPILLOMAVIRUS

More information about the Gardasil vaccine can be found on the Web site http://www.gardasil.com.

important to keep the following things in mind before and after you get the HPV vaccine:

- Although the vaccine protects against HPV types 6, 11, 16, and 18, the vaccine does not protect against all the types of HPV that cause cervical cancer.
- Although the vaccine protects against the HPV types that cause 90 percent of genital warts, it does not protect against all the HPV types that cause genital warts.

- While the vaccine protects against four major HPV types, it does not prevent other sexually transmitted infections.
- Girls and women who get the vaccine after they have acquired some of the HPV types will not get the full benefit of the vaccine, but they will still be protected from the HPV types they have not yet acquired.

The vaccine can be a great tool in preventing some cervical cancers and genital warts in many young women. And another HPV vaccine that would target two types of cervical cancer is in development. Learning more about the vaccine that's available now is a great step in looking after your health. (A vaccine that could protect males from some HPV-related conditions is being studied now, too. Hopefully, in the future, boys will have a safe, effective vaccine that can give them the kind of protection Gardasil can give girls and women.)

Condoms Offer Limited, but Valuable Protection

Condoms, also known as rubbers, offer protection against the spread of STDs. They also help prevent unplanned pregnancies. To do both effectively, condoms must be used every time a couple has sex. They must also be worn correctly. Widely available, condoms are inexpensive. They can be purchased or obtained at grocery, drug, and convenience stores; STD and health clinics; and some public restrooms. They are often offered for free at Planned Parenthood branches.

Condoms offer only limited protection from HPV. This is because condoms cannot cover pubic skin, a frequent site for genital warts. The only way to completely avoid HPV is to not have sex. Even spermicides like nonoxynol-9 are not effective for reducing the spread of HPV. If you notice any broken skin, unusual bumps, sores, or raised areas on you or your partner, don't have sex until a doctor determines the cause. Even though condoms cannot protect you fully from HPV, it is still a smart, sensible choice to use condoms. Remember, they can protect the areas of your genitals that are covered by the condom. They are also extremely effective, if used properly, at preventing unplanned pregnancies and many STDs.

A note on nonoxynol-9: It kills sperm and is the active ingredient in most over-the-counter spermicides. But nonoxynol-9 does NOT protect you from contracting the HIV virus (which causes AIDS) or other sexually transmitted diseases like gonorrhea or chlamydia. And while nonoxynol-9 can be used alone in cream or gel form, it is also used as a spermicide within condoms. There is also no evidence that condoms lubricated with nonoxynol-9 are any more effective in preventing pregnancy or infection than condoms lubricated with silicone, according to the World Health Organization (WHO). Last, frequent use of vaginal contraceptives with nonoxynol-9 can cause vaginal irritation and lesions (small cuts) in the vaginal wall, which can actually increase the likelihood of HIV infection. For all these reasons, many members of the medical community advise against the use of nonoxynol-9 as a means of birth control.

Condom Options

There are three types of condoms: latex, animal skin, and polyurethane. Latex condoms protect you against STDs. Polyurethane condoms also reduce the risk of infections, although studies show that polyurethane condoms are not as effective in protecting against pregnancy and sexually transmitted diseases. Condoms made from animal skin do not protect against disease. This is because viruses and bacteria can easily pass through animal tissue. Polyurethane condoms are available for males and females. Polyurethane condoms can be used with oil- and water-based medications or lubricants, although they are sometimes more expensive than latex condoms.

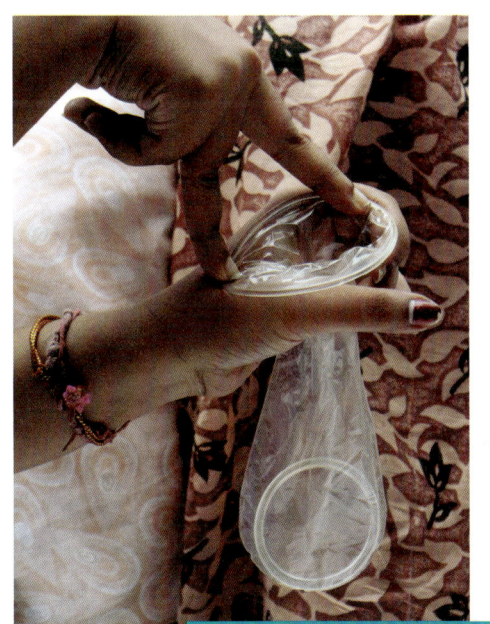

The Female Condom

A relatively new and highly effective barrier against pregnancy and sexually transmitted

The female condom is an effective barrier to pregnancy and sexually transmitted diseases.

diseases, the female condom is a plastic pouch with rings at each end that hold it in place comfortably. The outer ring remains outside the vagina, partly covering the labia, while the inner ring fits snugly inside. The female condom can be inserted up to several hours before a female has sex. It must be changed after each sexual encounter.

Oral Sex

Many people think oral sex (mouth to penis, or mouth to clitoris or vulva) is safer than intercourse (penis to vagina) when it comes to the spread of STDs. This is not true. STDs can be spread easily during oral sex, although male condoms provide a shield from transmission of some STDs.

Another important barrier is a dental dam. A small latex square, the dental dam is placed over the clitoris, vaginal opening, and labia to prevent any exchange of bodily fluids during oral sex.

Abstinence Is Not a Dirty Word

Although most teens would like to believe that nothing unexpected will happen when they have sex, the truth is that you and your partner take risks by becoming sexually active. You may put pressure on yourself to have sex because you think that all of your friends are "doing it." Believe it or not, many teens are choosing to abstain from—not engage in—sexual activity until they're older. This takes the pressure off sexual activity and allows time to set limits.

HOW CAN HUMAN PAPILLOMAVIRUS BE PREVENTED?

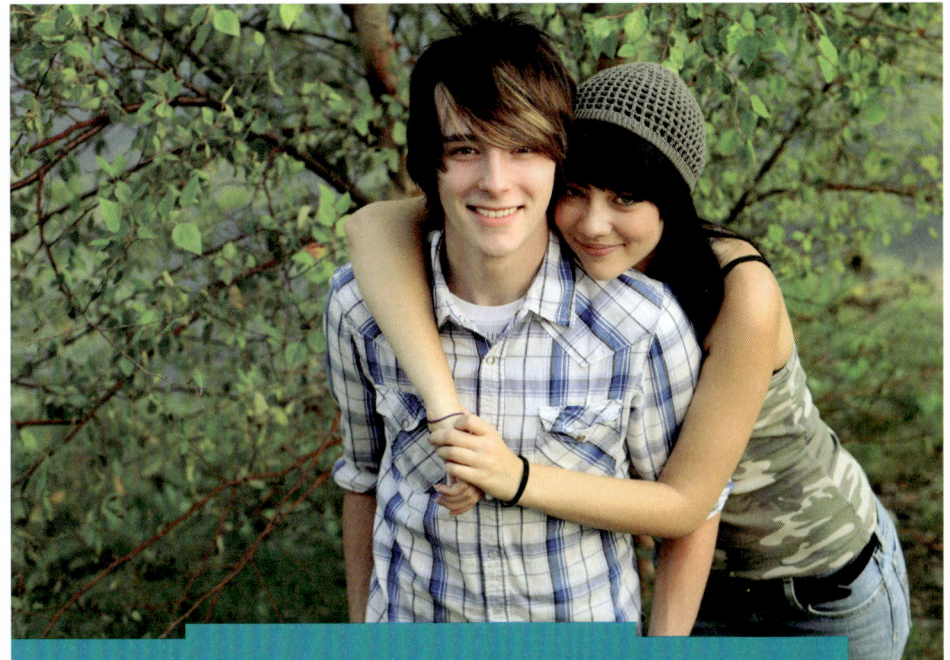

The surest way to prevent pregnancy and sexually transmitted diseases is abstinence. For couples who choose abstinence, there are still many other ways to show affection for one another.

You can still show affection and respect for each other by spending time talking, hugging, kissing, holding hands, and sharing common interests in sports, music, or other favorite activities.

Regular Checkups and Pap Smears Are Important

Because it is easy to get and spread HPV, it is important to get checked regularly. If you develop HPV, your risk of developing

A nurse performs a Pap test on a patient. Yearly Pap smears are an important part of preventing cervical cancer or at least catching it in its early stages.

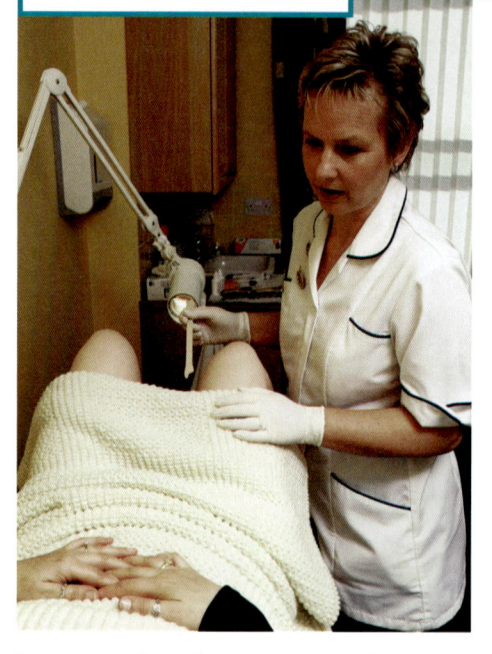

cancer of the cervix, anus, or penis can increase. All sexually active teens (male or female) and women should have yearly physicals, including screenings for sexually transmitted diseases. If you have an abnormal Pap smear, be sure to repeat the test as often as your doctor advises. If Pap smears are done annually, the chances are good that any cancer can be completely prevented or caught early, saving your life.

In addition to a Pap smear, your doctor may also do an HPV test. An HPV test is either conducted at the same time as a Pap smear or after a Pap smear with questionable results. Initial studies show that HPV tests are even better at detecting the presence of HPV than Pap smears and that they can ultimately better detect women at risk for cervical cancer so that these women can get the early treatment that they need.

Despite the Pap smear and HPV test's effectiveness and availability, a number of women still develop and die from cervical cancer. Elderly and low-income women often lack access to affordable screenings. Younger women may not realize the importance of regular testing. Sometimes, other cultural or social issues keep girls and women from getting the medical care that they need. You can talk to your parents if you have concerns or feel that you need to see a doctor. Your school nurse can also answer questions you may have. The bottom line on Pap smears and HPV tests is that all females should have them because they prevent needless deaths.

Chapter four

WHAT ARE THE TREATMENT OPTIONS FOR HUMAN PAPILLOMAVIRUS?

Several medications that are used to treat genital warts are available by prescription only and can be easily applied to any external genital warts by the patient. They offer effective relief for any itching, bleeding, or other discomforts warts cause. Medications designed to treat warts on the hands or feet will not work on genital warts and should not be used. The treatments described here only get rid of the symptoms; they do not cure HPV or genital warts. Following any treatment, HPV remains in the body. Symptoms can reappear, especially during the first year or so after diagnosis. In many cases, the body's immune system fights HPV so that it causes no further symptoms.

Liquids, Creams, and Gels

- **Podofilox:** Inexpensive and safe, this medication comes in a liquid or gel that can be applied by the patient to his or her external genital warts. Podofilox should not be used if you are pregnant.
- **Imiquimod cream:** Specially designed to treat external genital warts, including those around the anus, this medication is also safe and easy to apply. Imiquimod stimulates the body's immune system to help fight HPV. This is another cream that should not be used when pregnant.

Other topical ointments and chemicals must be applied in your doctor's office. These chemicals may cause some pain, burning, and irritation since each destroys the tissue affected by genital warts.

- **Podophyllin or podophyllotoxin:** This chemical is derived from a natural plant extract. It must remain on the infected area from one to four hours. Afterward, it is completely washed off and then reapplied weekly for up to six weeks. Extreme care must be taken with podophyllin because it may burn or scar the skin surrounding the genital warts. It isn't recommended if you are pregnant.
- **Trichloroacetic acid, or TCA:** Another chemical alternative that must be applied to warts in the doctor's office or in a clinic. TCA is a drug that causes genital warts to clot or solidify and is used only to treat small internal or external

> A syringe is filled with an interferon, an antiviral drug. The drug increases the activity of certain white blood cells and can be an effective treatment for HPV.

genital wart clusters. TCA is an acceptable treatment during pregnancy.

- **Fluorouracil:** This is a unique chemical that interferes with the DNA synthesis of HPV. Also a topical ointment, Fluorouracil causes a great deal of irritation but is useful in the treatment of vaginal (internal) and vulvar (external) genital warts.
- **Interferons, or IFNs:** These drugs are used only after other methods of wart removal have failed. Interferons are antiviral drugs that are injected directly into the wart, sometimes as often as three times per week. IFNs may cause many side effects; other treatments eliminate warts as well or better.

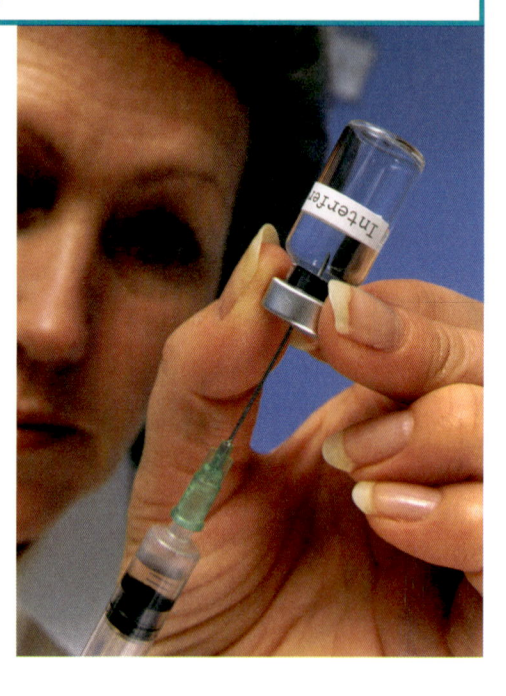

Physical Methods of Wart Removal

Although some of the following wart removal therapies may be painful, your doctor will perform them if other remedies fail. All methods described in this section require anesthesia.

- **Cryotherapy:** This "freezing" method involves the removal of genital warts using liquid nitrogen. This method destroys warts and the immediate surrounding area. Cryotherapy normally takes several visits to your doctor over the course of many weeks and is a safe method to choose if pregnant.
- **Laser surgery or therapy:** A high-intensity light is used to remove warts from the genitals or other areas of the body. This removal method is effective for sparing other healthy surrounding tissue and is safe if pregnant. Only specially trained doctors can perform laser procedures.
- **Electrosurgery:** This method involves the use of high-frequency currents to destroy interior tissue affected by genital warts. This may be an effective treatment option for internal cervical venereal warts. Usually, electrosurgery is even more effective for eliminating venereal warts than laser surgery or cryotherapy.
- **Surgical excision:** Surgery is sometimes preferred over other methods simply because it tends to cause less overall pain and allows for improved healing. Surgical removal of internal venereal warts is a choice made by doctors when warts are extensive.

Other Important Considerations

You may be told not to have sex until the treated areas have completely healed. Your partner also should be treated, even if he or she has no symptoms. Do not share or swap medications with your partner.

Ten Great Questions to Ask Your Doctor

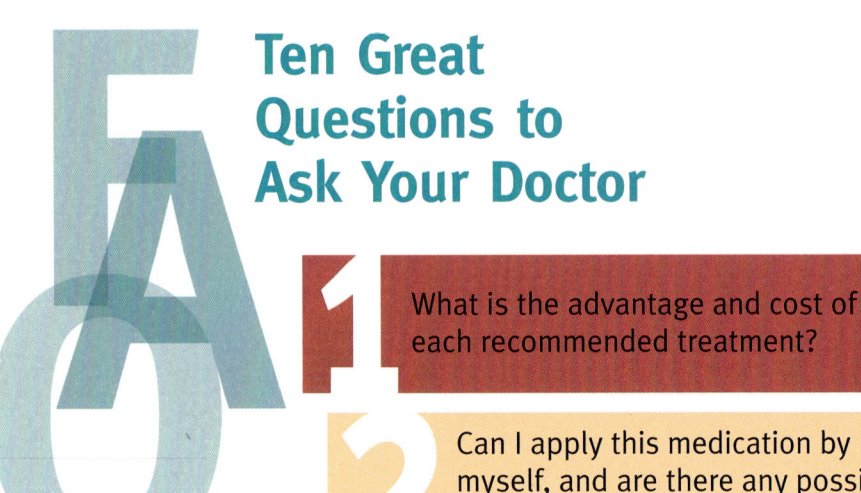

1. What is the advantage and cost of each recommended treatment?

2. Can I apply this medication by myself, and are there any possible side effects of this medication?

3. What will I need to do if any itching, bleeding, or pain occurs following treatment?

4. Will I need more than one treatment?

5. What do I need to do if the warts come back?

6. Can you tell me more about the Pap smear (or anal Pap smear) test? Do I need a Pap smear at this time?

7. Are there any precautions I should take if I am pregnant?

WHAT ARE THE TREATMENT OPTIONS FOR HUMAN PAPILLOMAVIRUS?

8 When will I need to return for any additional treatment or follow-up visits?

9 Does having HPV make me more vulnerable to other STDs?

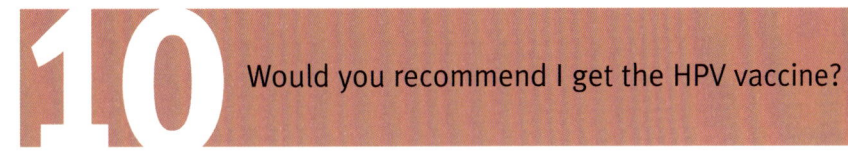

10 Would you recommend I get the HPV vaccine?

Chapter five

WHAT IS THE CONNECTION BETWEEN HUMAN PAPILLOMAVIRUS AND CERVICAL CANCER?

While only a small number of females with an HPV infection will develop cervical cancer, medical researchers now know that particular strains of HPV, such as 16, 18, 31, 33, and 45, are responsible for approximately 99 percent of all cervical cancers.

Cervical cancer is considered a public health threat. The number of cervical cancer cases diagnosed yearly in the United States is 14,500; of these, 4,800 end in death. Many or all of these deaths are preventable. With early diagnosis and treatment of cervical cell changes, lives can be saved.

Researchers think that most of these cervical cancers develop when viruses harm the genes (the body's blueprint for growth and function) that tell the body to produce the

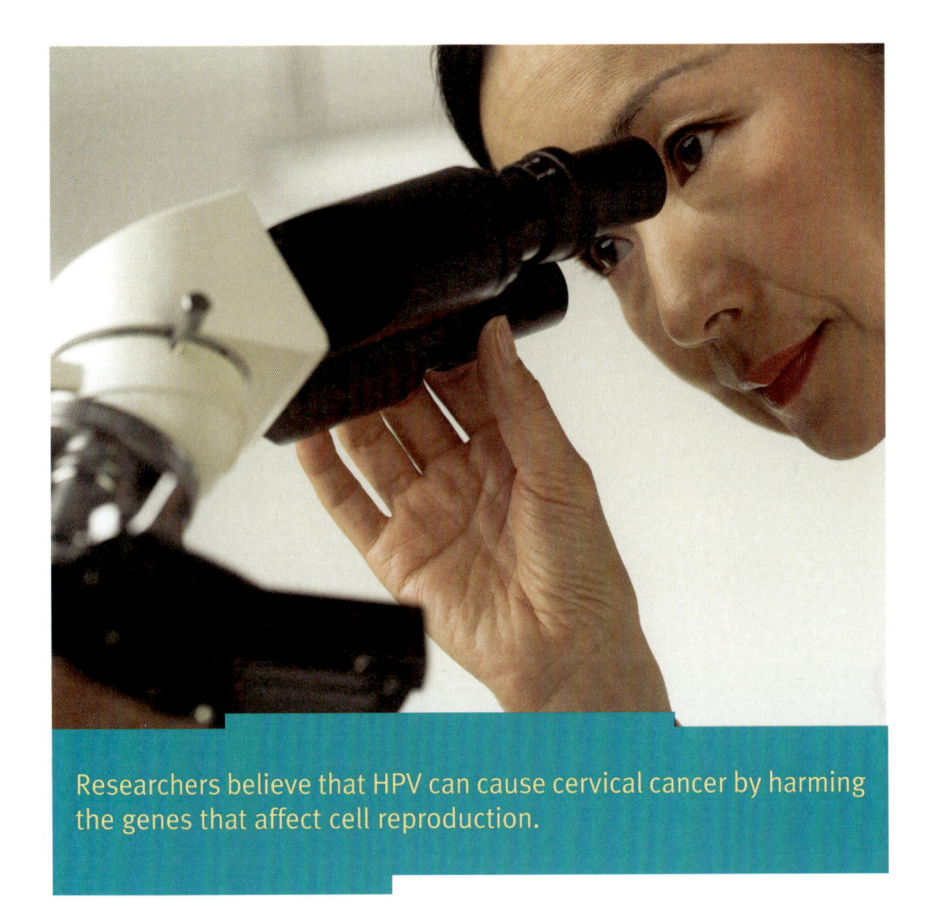

WHAT IS THE CONNECTION BETWEEN HUMAN PAPILLOMAVIRUS AND CERVICAL CANCER?

Researchers believe that HPV can cause cervical cancer by harming the genes that affect cell reproduction.

right number of normal cells. Because of the virus, the body produces too many abnormal cells.

While cervical cancer can take years to develop, doctors in the United States are seeing cases in which precancerous cervical changes occur much more quickly. How the body reacts to HPV depends on many things: the particular strains in a person's body, the ability of the immune system to fight off HPV, and whether or not the person has other risk factors that can make it easier to contract HPV or develop cervical cancer.

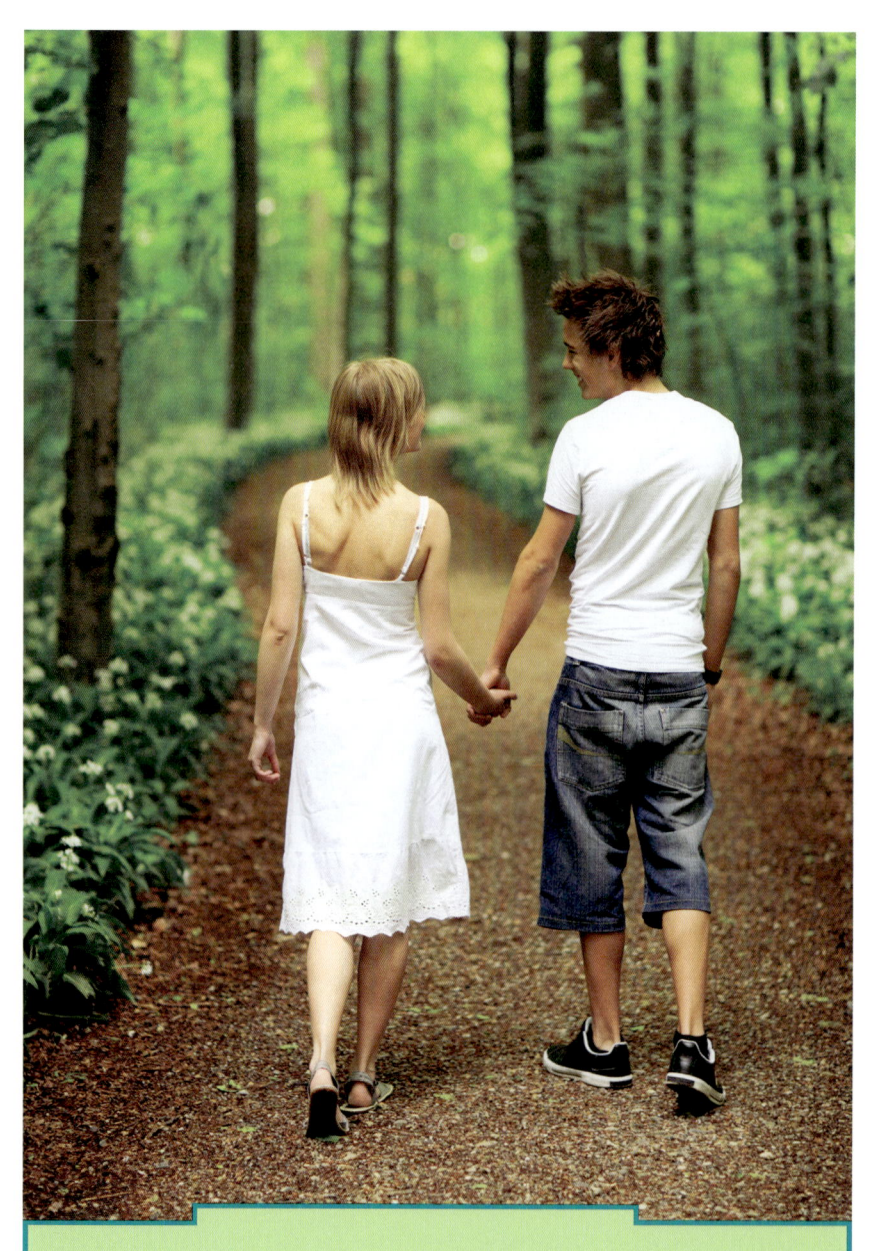

36 FREQUENTLY ASKED QUESTIONS ABOUT HUMAN PAPILLOMAVIRUS

To lower your risk of contracting HPV, limit the number of people you have sex with, avoid sex with high-risk partners, and use a condom if you do have sex.

Lowering Your Risk

While the subject of HPV and cervical cancer may be frightening, there are many simple steps you can take to minimize your risk if you are a girl:

- Put off sex until the age of twenty-one or after. Abstaining from sex until you're in your twenties dramatically cuts your chances of developing cervical HPV infection and later cancer. It also allows your cervix to develop fully so it is less vulnerable to infection. Females who have sex before the age of sixteen are at greater risk for cervical cancer.
- Limit the number of people you have sex with. If your partner has had sex with many people, your risk of HPV infection increases. Choose someone who has had fewer partners and is willing to have sex only with you.
- Insist that your partner always use a condom every time you have sex. Using a condom limits your exposure to other STDs and decreases potential stress on the body's immune system. Also, whatever type of birth control you choose, it should offer dual protection. First, it should protect against pregnancy. But second—and just as important—it should protect against potentially deadly sexually transmitted diseases like the HIV virus (which causes AIDS) as well as gonorrhea, chlamydia, and others.
- Avoid sex with high-risk partners. A high-risk partner is someone who has had many partners, has a history of STD infection or partners with that history, or began having sex earlier than age sixteen.

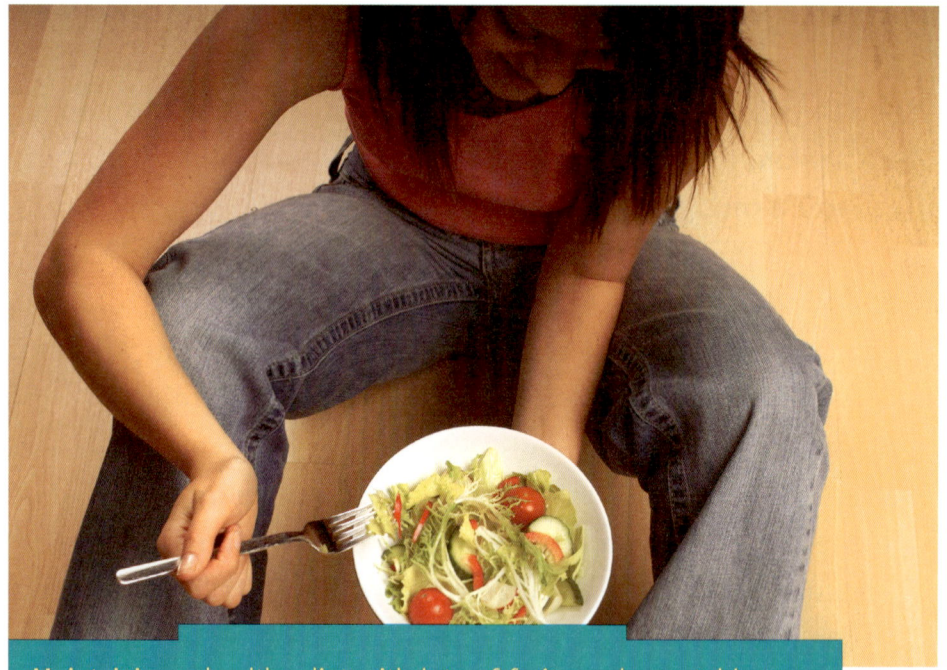

Maintaining a healthy diet with lots of fruits and vegetables can boost your immune system and help you fight off HPV if you are exposed.

- Avoid smoking. Research suggests that because smoking stresses the body's immune system, it makes it easier to become infected with HPV.
- Avoid consumption of alcohol. Research has proven that there is a definitive connection between cervical cancer and high levels of alcohol consumption.
- Maintain a level of wellness. Low levels of vitamin A, vitamin C, folic acid, and beta-carotene could contribute to the development of cervical cancer. Adhering to a healthy diet and proper hydration, combined with other healthy life

choices, helps keep your immune system in shape, too. A healthy immune system is your best defense against HPV or any STD infection.

➤ Follow your doctor's advice about how often Pap smears should be done. (The American Cancer Society recommends yearly Pap smears and pelvic exams for all sexually active females and any woman over the age of eighteen.) Be especially alert for any symptoms of genital warts, vaginal discharge, or changes in your period.

Colposcopy

When doctors want a better look at the tissue in your cervix following an abnormal Pap smear, they may use a special magnifying lens with a light attached to it, called a colposcope. During the examination, certain staining liquids, such as acetic acid or Lougal's iodine, are applied to the cervix to identify cancerous lesions. The colposcopy procedure can help identify changes in cervical cells, abnormal groups of cells on the cervix, or the development of cancer. In many circumstances, depending on the results of the colposcopy test, your doctor may then suggest that you undergo a test called a biopsy.

Biopsy

If a closer exam is needed to see these cellular changes, your doctor may request a biopsy. During a biopsy, a small bit of cervical tissue (cells from the inside of the cervix) is removed and examined in a pathology lab. This test takes less than fifteen minutes and is practically painless (some patients experience

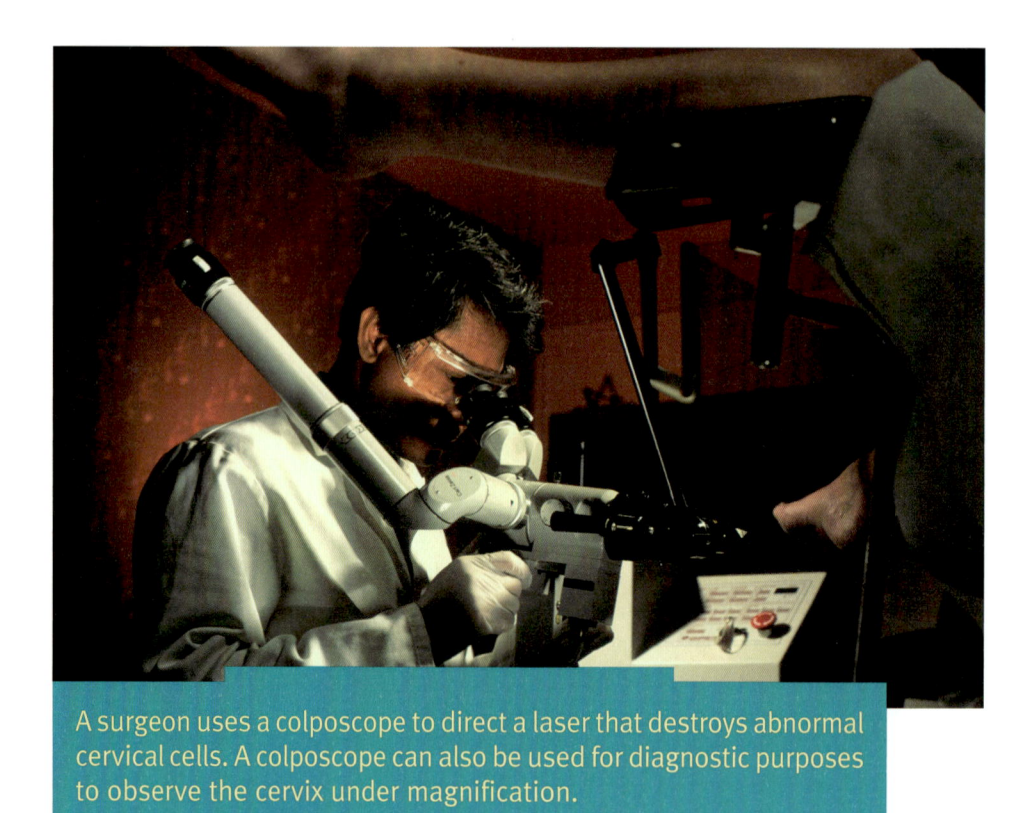

A surgeon uses a colposcope to direct a laser that destroys abnormal cervical cells. A colposcope can also be used for diagnostic purposes to observe the cervix under magnification.

slight cramping or bleeding afterward). A biopsy test allows your doctor the ability to analyze the exact cells that are causing abnormalities in the Pap smear results.

Hybrid Capture II HPV Test

This test is intended to help doctors locate which strains of HPV a female has in her body. The HPV test is used after repeated Pap smears have shown cervical cell abnormalities. It can help identify a female's chances of developing cervical cancer by showing whether she has a strain of HPV that is more likely to cause cancer later. This allows doctors to watch the situation carefully and treat cervical changes before any cancer develops.

A positive HPV test does not mean that you have cervical cancer. It simply means that you've been infected with HPV. Most females with HPV don't develop cancer, but knowing and understanding your risk can help you make better decisions about your health.

Dysplasia

Dysplasia is the medical word that describes changes in the cells of the cervix. These changes happen before any cancer appears and include variations in the shapes of the cells on the surface of the cervix. Doctors classify dysplasia as mild, moderate, or severe, depending on the abnormality seen when the cells are examined.

Dysplasia does not necessarily develop into cervical cancer; your doctor may suggest monitoring the cell changes closely with more frequent testing, or he or she may treat the condition if it is moderate or severe. If your dysplasia is mild, it may go away on its own.

Many females with dysplasia never have any symptoms or discomfort, but any changes in your period, abdominal pain, or discharge from your vagina should be reported to your doctor immediately.

Heavy bleeding, longer than normal periods, bleeding after sex, vaginal discharge that smells, fatigue, and pain are some of the symptoms signaling cervical cancer. They may not appear until the later stages of the disease and should never be ignored.

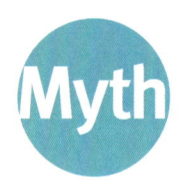

Myths and Facts

Myth **My girlfriend and I always use condoms. We don't worry about human papillomavirus (HPV) because condoms protect us.** **Fact** ➔ Condoms do not always protect you against getting or giving HPV. Because the virus is passed through skin-to-skin contact, as well as through fluids, any skin that is not covered by a condom is at risk of HPV transmission. On the other hand, using condoms has been shown to reduce a female's chances of getting cervical cancer from HPV later. Condoms also protect against pregnancy and HIV/AIDS.

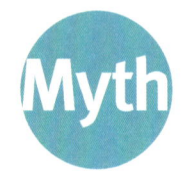

Myth **Cervical cancer is not preventable.** **Fact** ➔ Cervical cancer can often be prevented. We know that high-risk strains of HPV are the cause of almost all cases of cervical cancer. Females who are at risk for cervical cancer can be tested to see which strain of HPV they have. Doctors can keep a close eye on a patient if she is found to have a high-risk strain in her body.

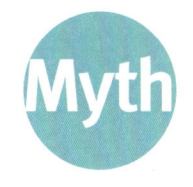

Myth **If you have HPV, you will get cervical/penile/anal cancer.** **Fact** ⇒ We do know that there is a link between HPV and these cancers. However, getting HPV is not the equivalent of a death sentence. Cervical cancer is relatively rare. Penile and anal cancers are even less common than cervical cancer. Once you are infected, the symptoms of HPV infection usually go away in a few months without any problems. Studies show that 70 percent of new HPV infections in young women disappear within one year, and as many as 91 percent disappear within two years. However, it's important to see your gynecologist or doctor regularly.

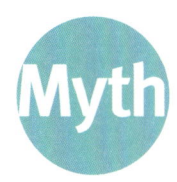

Myth **Only girls who sleep around (or whose boyfriends are unfaithful) are at risk of getting HPV.** **Fact** ⇒ Almost eight out of ten sexually active people will get HPV by the age of fifty. HPV is the most common sexually transmitted infection in the United States. Both males and females can get HPV; and both males and females can get cancers later in life as a result of HPV infection.

Myth

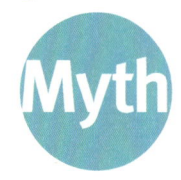

If my Pap smears are always normal, I don't need to worry about having or getting STDs. **Fact**

A Pap smear does not test for the presence of HPV or other STDs. A Pap smear can tell your doctor if there are abnormal cell changes in your cervix—an early sign of cervical cancer. To find out whether you have an STD, you must ask your doctor for a test specific to that STD. Even if your Pap smears are normal, one of the best precautions against STD infection is the use of condoms during sex. Condoms cannot, however, prevent all infections.

Chapter Six

WHAT IS THE CONNECTION BETWEEN HUMAN PAPILLOMAVIRUS AND PENILE AND ANAL CANCERS?

In addition to causing cervical and other cancers in women, certain high-risk strains of human papillomavirus (HPV)—strains 16, 18, 31, 33, and 45—can also lead to cancer of the penis or anus in males.

Anal cancers are relatively rare but appear to be on the rise. Females are more likely to have cancers in the inner part of the anus (the anal canal). Males tend to get anal tumors on the outside of the anus. Although penile and anal cancers are uncommon, understanding their connection to HPV, as well as to other known risk factors, can help you make important decisions about your sexual habits and health.

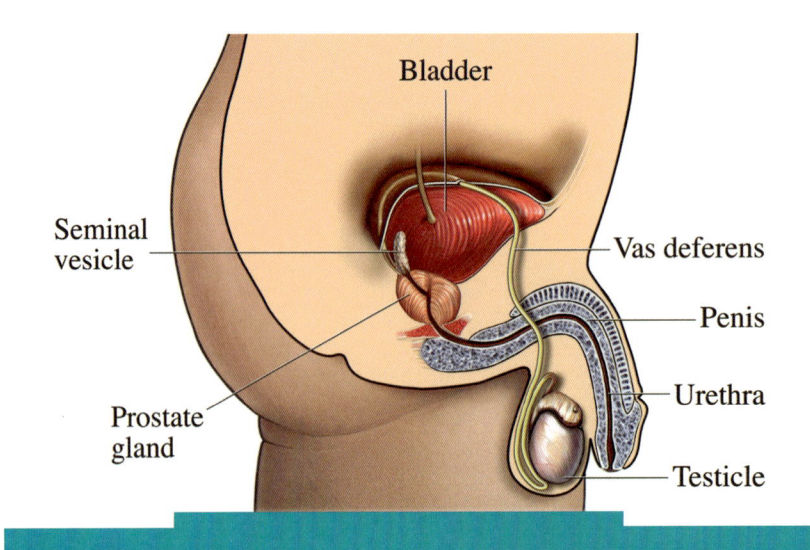

Above is a diagram of the male reproductive system.

Penile Cells and Cancer

Each part of the penis is made up of various kinds of cells that form the skin, nerves, muscle, and the three small chambers that contain an extensive web of blood vessels and tissue. A different type of cancer could invade each of these groups. This is significant because where a particular cancer grows helps doctors know how it can impact a male's health, how quickly it is likely to spread, and the best methods for treating it.

Most cancers of the penis—about 95 percent—result from flat, scaly skin cells known as squamous cells. Squamous cell cancers can find a home anywhere on the penis, but they usually settle on either the glans (the tip of the penis) or the foreskin (the retractable covering that hoods the glans) unless a male has been

WHAT IS THE CONNECTION BETWEEN HUMAN PAPILLOMAVIRUS AND PENILE AND ANAL CANCERS?

circumcised (had his foreskin surgically removed). These cancers generally develop quite slowly and are curable if found early.

Adenocarcinoma of the penis is a rare type of squamous cell cancer that advances from the sweat glands found in penile skin. When adenocarcinoma occurs in the skin of the penis, it is called Paget's disease. These cancer cells initially spread in the skin. At later stages, these cells develop in the lymph nodes (tiny groups of disease-fighting cells that are part of the body's immune system).

Another infrequent kind of squamous cell cancer occurs in both males and females. Often called Bushke-Lowenstein tumor, this cancer can be found on the genitals of males and females as well as on the skin, or inside the anus, mouth, or larynx. It closely resembles noncancerous genital warts and rarely spreads to other parts of the body.

Other penile cancers can form from the cells that manufacture your skin's color or pigment. Known as melanomas, these cancers normally appear on skin that has been repeatedly exposed to sunlight or has been repeatedly sunburned. Melanomas may also develop on the penis or in other less exposed areas and are responsible for only about 2 percent of penile cancers. Although this is a very small number, melanomas can grow and spread very quickly, making them an aggressive, and sometimes deadly, form of cancer.

Sarcomas are cancers that evolve from penile muscle cells, blood vessel cells, or the cells of other membranes of the penis. They constitute about 1 percent of all cancers of the penis.

Basal cell cancers also normally grow on sun-exposed portions of the body. Unlike melanomas, these cancers develop slowly

A cervical Pap smear slide shows normal squamous epithelial cells, the cells that make up the outer wall of the cervix.

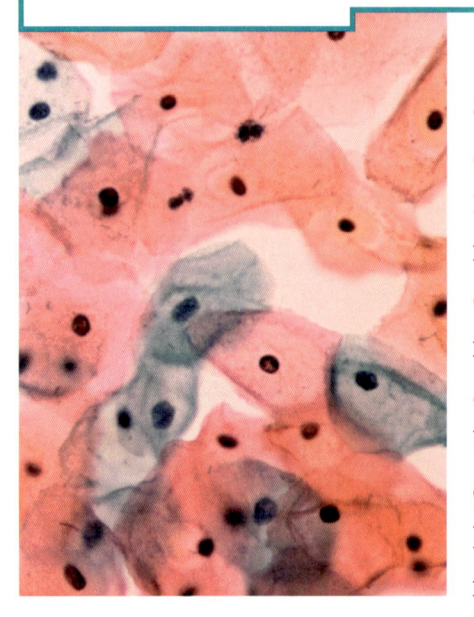

and do not often spread to other areas. They account for less than 2 percent of penile cancers. A factor that greatly influences the onset and outcome of treatment is waiting too long. The earlier and more quickly you respond by getting medical attention, the greater your chances of staying healthy. See your doctor at the first signs of any abnormality.

Squamous Cell Cancers and Dysplasia

Squamous cancers usually develop after precancerous changes in the cells of penile tissue occur. Referred to by doctors as dysplasia or penile intraepithelial neoplasia, these precancerous changes happen slowly and involve only cells on the top layer of the penile skin.

A male with precancerous dysplasia may develop one or many warts, which can range from being virtually invisible to appearing like a miniature head of cauliflower. Other unusual growths or irritated sections of skin can also indicate dysplasia. These changes most often occur on the glans or foreskin but may also happen along the shaft of the penis. It is important to remember that, although many types of warts are benign (not cancerous), any change in the appearance of the penis should be immediately examined by a doctor.

A Wide Array of Symptoms

Symptoms of penile cancer vary. They include painless ulcers on the glans, foreskin, or shaft. A reddish, velvety rash on the penis; sores; blisters; crusty or patchy white areas; a thickening of the skin; an enduring, smelly discharge from under the foreskin; or bleeding, as well as swollen lymph nodes in and around the groin, can also signal cancer. Swelling at the end of the penis or in the groin is an additional signal that should not be ignored. Symptoms that develop beneath the foreskin may be difficult to see until it is retracted. In some instances, a male may have no symptoms until the cancer has advanced to later stages.

Diagnosing Penile Cancers

The first step in detecting any cancer involves a thorough inspection of the penis by a doctor. When abnormalities are found, a biopsy is done to confirm the presence and type of cancer. The biopsied tissue is carefully checked in a pathology lab. This removed tissue can also reveal at which stage the cancer has been found and what future tests need to be conducted.

The doctor may perform an ultrasound, a computed tomography scan (CT scan), or a magnetic resonance imaging test (MRI). Each of these allow the doctor to see the cancer quickly, painlessly, and fully, with virtually no discomfort to the patient. All of these tests provide doctors with additional information they must have to effectively treat any cancer. The treatment a

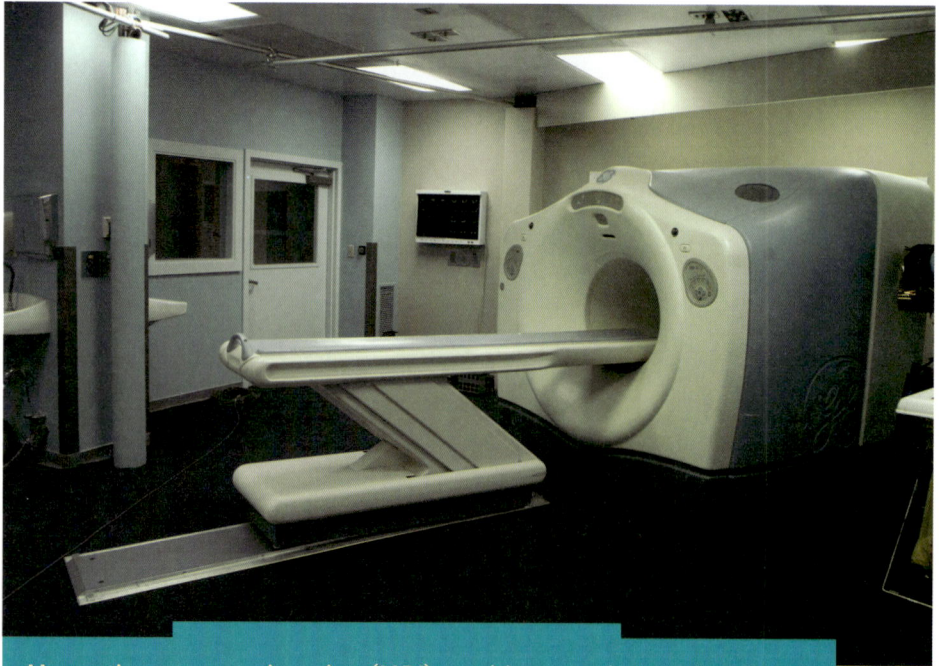

Magnetic resonance imaging (MRI) machines can be used to detect cancers or provide necessary information to doctors treating cancer patients.

patient receives depends on the type of cancer, its stage of development, and its location, as well as other factors.

Risk Factors for Penile Cancer

Risk factors for penile cancer include the following:

- **HPV infection:** This disease is seen as a preventable risk factor for penile and anal cancer. Currently, there is no test a male can take to detect HPV infection, such as the Hybrid Capture II HPV test for females. Young men can reduce the risk of HPV infection by putting off having sex until later in life, reducing the number of sex partners, using condoms to practice safe sex, not smoking, reducing stress on the immune system by not contracting other STDs, eating healthily, and getting adequate exercise and rest. Also, keeping the area under the foreskin clean and free of infection is another suggestion. (Avoid a buildup of smegma, an oily, sometimes cheeselike substance that can build up under the foreskin if the male is not careful about keeping that area clean.)

- **Smoking:** Researchers have noticed a correlation between cancer development and smoking. They believe that smoking alters the DNA of penile cells and contributes to the development of cancerous cells, especially in males who also have HPV in their bodies.
- **Phimosis:** A condition in which the foreskin becomes hard to pull back. Phimosis may lead to too much smegma around the tip of the penis, making it harder to keep clean and raising possible cancer risks.
- **Psoriasis, drug, and light interaction:** According to information provided by the American Cancer Society, males with the skin condition known as psoriasis who are treated with ultraviolet light and/or a drug called Psorafen tend to have higher levels of penile cancer.

Anal Cancer

The anus is actually part of an intricate system designed to rid the body of waste. It is found at the lowest end of your large intestine. Known as the rectum, this portion of the intestine serves as the collection point for waste (feces) that passes out of the anal opening. The uppermost part of the large intestine is called the colon.

Most cancers of the anus develop from squamous cells. Called squamous cell carcinomas, these cancers begin on the surface of anal skin. Some spread beyond the surface and attack surrounding tissues. Other anal cancers include adenocarcinomas. These often develop in glands underneath the skin. Glands are cells, groups of cells, or organs of the body that produce and secrete fluids such as mucus or sweat. Basal cell cancers and melanomas can also develop in or on anal tissue, but this is uncommon.

Risk Factors for Anal Cancer

Risk factors for anal cancer include the following:

- **HPV infection:** HPV can be spread through anal (as well as vaginal or oral) sex. Some of the warts produced by certain strains of HPV can become cancerous.
- **Smoking:** According to the American Cancer Society, if you smoke, you are eight times more likely than a nonsmoker to suffer from cancer of the anus.
- **Reduced immunity:** A compromised immune system increases your chances of developing anal cancer. This includes people with HIV, the virus that causes AIDS, or those who have had organ transplants and need to take medications to prevent organ rejection.
- **Engaging in high-risk sexual activity:** Research suggests that increased high-risk sexual activities such as receptive

WHAT IS THE CONNECTION BETWEEN HUMAN PAPILLOMAVIRUS AND PENILE AND ANAL CANCERS?

> Smoking cigarettes increases your risk of developing cancer, including anal cancer, which, according to the American Cancer Society, you are eight times more likely to contract if you smoke.

anal sex could possibly increase a person's chances of developing anal cancer.

Symptoms of Anal Cancer

Some of the symptoms of anal cancer include:

- Pain in your anal area
- Anal itching
- Straining during bowel movements
- A change in the frequency of your bowel movements
- Any swelling in the anal or groin areas
- Anal discharge

Diagnosing Anal Cancer

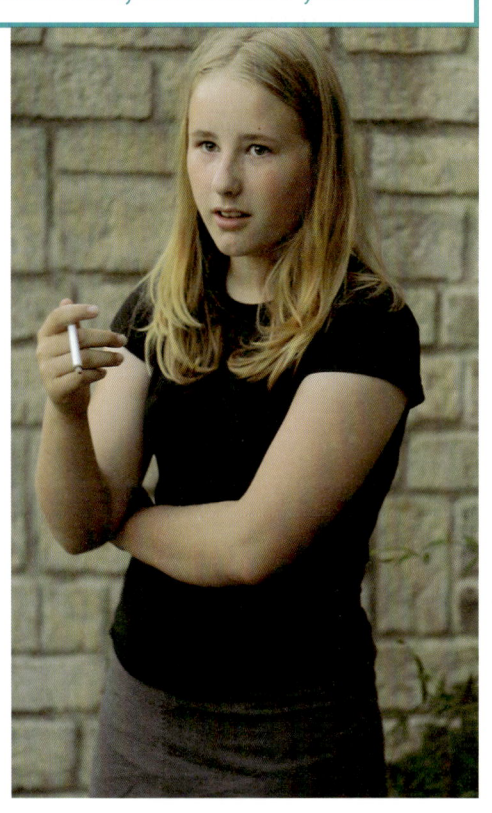

For both males and females, anal cancer is sometimes found following a physical exam or a rectal exam in which the doctor feels the inside of the anus and rectum for any signs of abnormality, such as tissue masses, polyps (projection growths), or abscesses (tissues that produce mucus). Similar to the screening tests for cervical cancer in females, a swab is often inserted into the anal canal to collect a cell sample. The sample is then sent to a pathology lab for further examination and testing. Medical staff refers to this test as an anal Pap smear.

If any abnormal growth is detected, your doctor may recommend any of several procedures that allow him or her to view anal tissue. An anoscopy (similar to a colposcopy where a lighted instrument assists doctors in viewing interior tissues), a biopsy, or an examination of swollen lymph nodes may follow this detection. If cancer is found, tests such as CT scans or ultrasound can help determine its type and stage of development.

It's important to remember that both males and females may get anal cancer. Anal cancer is rare and usually curable if found early, and regular checkups are the key to early detection. Once found, anal cancer is usually treated with a combination of radiation and chemotherapy—both are treatments to stop cancerous cells from reproducing.

As with cervical and penile cancers, it is best to understand your risk factors, particularly those connected with the spread of HPV, so you can make healthy decisions.

Glossary

abnormal In a Pap smear, results may be defined as abnormal or positive, meaning that the results have tested positive for a certain amount of inflamed, irritated, or abnormal cells or cellular changes.

abstinence Not having sex or not engaging in certain other sexual activities.

active Describes a phase of a disease in which there are symptoms or infectious activity.

anus The bodily opening from the rectum to the outside of the body.

benign Noncancerous.

biopsy The clinical process of removing a tiny tissue sample from inside the body for closer, microscopic examination.

cancer A disease marked by abnormal cell growth. Some cancer types spread deeply into tissues while others remain in one area.

cervix The narrow portion of the uterus that opens into the vagina.

colposcopy A special examination that allows a closer inspection of the cervix. During a colposcopy procedure, a microscope called a colposcope is used to magnify the cervix. This helps the doctor look for visible signs of internal genital warts or an HPV infection.

condom A latex sheath that fits over the penis and helps prevent pregnancy and exposure to sexually transmitted diseases. Female condoms line the inside of the vagina and cover the outer labia.

dysplasia Medical term for cell changes that occur before cancer develops.

genital Referring to the penis, scrotum, or testes in males, and the labia, vagina, or clitoris in females.

genital wart A raised skin growth or bump that develops as a result of HPV infection. Genital warts can be very small and difficult to notice, or large, flat, and raised. They can appear singly or in clusters resembling cauliflower.

hormones Chemicals that regulate the body's growth and many of its functions.

human papillomavirus A group of viruses that can cause warts to develop on or inside the body, particularly in the genital area. Some strains of human papillomavirus also lead to certain types of cancers in males and females. Also called HPV.

inactive Describes a phase of a disease in which there are no symptoms or infectious activity. The infecting organism is present but dormant.

labia The outer lips or opening to the vagina.

latent HPV A period of inactivity for HPV, during which no symptoms may be apparent. Symptoms may reappear at any time.

Pap smear A procedure used by a doctor to check for abnormal cells in the cervix that could lead to cancer. A small amount

GLOSSARY

of tissue is swabbed from inside the vaginal area and sent to a pathology lab for further examination. Anal Pap smears can also be performed.

penis The external sex organ of a male.

precancerous This term is used to describe cells that may be on the way to becoming cancerous but are not yet truly cancerous.

STD A disease, such as HPV or AIDS, that is transmitted through sexual contact with an infected person; stands for sexually transmitted disease.

vagina Passage from a female's uterus or womb to the outside of the body.

virus A microorganism that invades and uses the cells of the body to reproduce itself.

For More Information

The American Cancer Society
1599 Clifton Road NE
Atlanta, GA 30329-4251
(800) ACS-2345 (227-2345)
Web site: http://www.cancer.org

> The Web site includes cancer resources, news, and information. Search for topics including cervical, penile, and anal cancers. Learn what's involved in treatment so you can make informed decisions. The Web site also offers links to an extensive support network for people with cancer, their friends, and their families.

The American Social Health Association (ASHA)
P.O. Box 13827
Research Triangle Park, NC 27713
(919) 361-8400
(800) 230-6039
Web site: http://www.ashast.org

> Confidential brochures on HPV, information on local support groups, and an online HPV chatroom are available from ASHA. To obtain brochures, call ASHA will also answer questions about HPV through e-mail, at hpvnet@ashastd.org

FOR MORE INFORMATION

Centers for Disease Control and Prevention (CDC)
1600 Clifton Road
Atlanta, GA 30333
National STD Hotline: (800) 227-8922
Web site: http://www.cdc.gov

> Information to address your health concerns, as well as scientific information on infectious diseases, is available through the Web site of the CDC. Educational and student resources for grades K–12 are also offered. The Web site features an easy-to-use index of infectious diseases, including sexually transmitted diseases.

National Cancer Institute
Public Inquiries Office
Building 31, Room 10A31
31 Center Drive MSC 2580
Bethesda, MD 20892-2580
(301) 435-3848
(800) 4-CANCER (442-6237)
Web site: http://www.nci.nih.gov

> The Web site offers a dictionary of cancer terms, a cancer drug dictionary, and general information about all types of cancers, their causes, prevention, screening, and treatments. There is also a section for Spanish speakers and access to cancer statistics and an annual report summarizing scientific data for the general public.

Planned Parenthood Federation of America
810 Seventh Avenue
New York, NY 10019
(212) 541-7800
(800) 230-PLAN (7526)
Web site: http://www.plannedparenthood.org

Planned Parenthood provides information about reproductive health and sexually transmitted diseases. The Web site includes an "Ask a Doctor" section. There is also a searchable database of medical service providers for those wishing to talk to a professional about HPV.

Web Sites

Due to the changing nature of Internet links, Rosen Publishing has developed an online list of Web sites related to the subject of this book. This site is updated regularly. Please use this link to access the list:

http://www.rosenlinks.com/faq/hupa

For Further Reading

Carter, Elizabeth. *Everything You Need to Know About Human Papillomavirus.* New York, NY: Rosen Publishing Group, 2001.

Haerens, Margaret, ed. *Sexually Transmitted Diseases.* Detroit, MI : Greenhaven Press, 2007.

Handley, Jody, and Joel Palefsky. *What Your Doctor May Not Tell You About HPV and Abnormal Pap Smears.* New York, NY: Warner Books, 2002.

Kolesnikow, Tassia. *Sexually Transmitted Diseases.* San Diego, CA: Lucent Books, 2004.

Index

A
abstinence, 24–25, 37
adenocarcinoma, 47, 52
anal cancer, 6, 26, 43, 45, 50, 51–54
anal Pap smear, 54
anoscopy, 54

B
basal cell cancers, 47–48, 52
biopsy, 13, 39–40, 49, 54
Bushke-Lowenstein tumor, 47

C
cervical cancer, 6, 17, 19, 20, 21, 26, 34–44, 45, 54
chlamydia, 16, 22, 37
colposcopy, 12, 39, 54
condoms, 21–24, 37, 42, 44, 51
cryotherapy, 31

D
dental dam, 24
dysplasia, 41–42, 48

E
electrosurgery, 31

F
fluorouracil, 30

G
Gardasil, 17–21
genital herpes, 16
genital warts, 6–8, 9–15, 17, 19, 20, 21, 22, 28–31, 39, 48–49
gonorrhea, 16, 22, 37

H
hepatitis B and C, 16
HIV/AIDS, 16, 22, 37, 52
human papillomavirus (HPV)
    diagnosing, 12–13
    explanation of, 6–8
    how it is spread, 9, 42
    myths and facts about, 42–44
    and pregnancy, 13–15
    prevention/lowering risk of, 16–27, 37–39
    symptoms of, 9–12
    treatment options for, 28–31
human papillomavirus (HPV) test, 26–27, 40–41, 50

I
imiquimod cream, 29
interferons (IFNs), 30

L
laser surgery/therapy, 31

INDEX

M
melanomas, 47, 52

N
National HPV and Cervical Cancer Prevention Resource Center, 8
nonoxynol-9, 22

O
oral sex, 9, 10, 24, 52

P
Pap smear, 10, 12, 19, 26–27, 39, 40, 44

penile cancer, 6, 26, 43, 45, 46–51, 54
podofilox, 29
podophyllin/podophyllotoxin, 29

S
sarcomas, 47
squamous cell cancers, 46, 47, 48–49, 52
surgical excision, 31
syphilis, 16

T
trichloroacetic acid (TCA), 29–30

Photo Credits

Cover © AJPhoto/Photo Researchers; p. 5 © James Cavallini/Photo Researchers; p. 7 © Custom Medical Stock Photo; pp. 11, 46 © Nucleus Medical Art, Inc./Getty Images; p. 13 © Saturn Stills/Photo Researchers; p. 14 © www.istockphoto.com/Bradley Bassitt; pp. 18, 23 © AFP/Getty Images; p. 25 © www.istockphoto.com/Tracy Whiteside; p. 26 © Mark Thomas/Photo Researchers; p. 30 © James King-Holmes/Photo Researchers; pp. 35, 36, 53 Shutterstock; p. 38 © www.istockphoto.com; p. 40 © Deep Light Productions/Photo Researchers; p. 48 © SPL/Photo Researchers; p. 50 © Getty Images.

Designer: Evelyn Horovicz; Editor: Peter Herman
Photo Researcher: Marty Levick